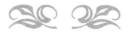

NATURE IMMERSION

Six Weeks to a Healthier and Stronger Mind, Body, and Spirit

Health and Lifestyle Transformation Coach

GHENE'T LEE-YONG

Nature Immersion

Cover and Interior Design by Transcendent Publishing.

ISBN: 978-1-0879-8020-1

strongereveryday1111.com,
Email Me ghenet.@strongereveryday1111.com

This workbook is not intended as a substitute for the medical advice of a medical professional. The reader is advised to regularly consult with a physician in matters relating to his/her health and particularly with respect to any symptoms that may require medical attention.

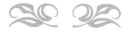

Dedication

I dedicate this workbook to my beautiful children, Kaitlynn and Bastion. Without whom I would not have had the imperative to change and to create a better life for them by first creating a better life for me. I am stronger everyday because of you.

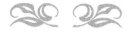

Introduction

Welcome to your journey to a healthier body and mind. Through Nature Immersion you can find peace and clarity while at the same time exercising your body. Nature immersion is best practiced outdoors. However, climate, physical ability, and timing might be an issue. I will show you how to practice these exercises both indoors and outside. When engaging in these activities I find early morning works best for me. However, I have done them on lunch break walks and in the late evening before the sun goes down. You can do these once a week to start slowly. When you feel more comfortable add more days. The best results come when practiced three to four times a week with a day or two for rest in between. The alternative exercises can be used on a day when you cannot go out, or for those who have limited mobility.

Enjoy your journey. Be strong and follow through to the end. Make sure to be gentle with yourself and most of all have fun, find peace, find clarity!

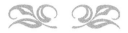

Week One - Centering

Welcome to the beginning of your journey to a mentally and physically healthier you. Through activities designed to get you outdoors and exploring the natural world you will discover a path that leads to fitness, mental dexterity and a deeper connection to nature. This week we will focus on centering yourself to the natural environment around you, oticing your space and where you fit in that space.

Walking Reflection- Observe the environment around you as you walk. Look at trees, notice squirrels, chipmunks, birds and even the flies or bees as they busily attend to their various errands. Observe natural objects. Rocks, sticks, moss, types of grass, the kind of soil in your area. Just take time to get to know the area where you choose to walk. Find a natural object to take back home with you. This will serve as a focal point for reflection or a connection to the outdoors when you are not able to get outside. **Alternative**- sit on your patio, back porch, backyard, or open window. Gently stretch as you do the above activity.

Walking Affirmation

The world around me is vast and confined at once
The natural world holds within it hidden kingdoms
of immeasurable beauty and complexity
I walk as one with this beauty wholly connected

Walking Record

Length of Time <u>Distance</u>

_____

Date and Time

_____

Journal Reflection- What did I see on my walk that I did not notice before? How did I feel before I went on my walk? Did I have any negative feelings or reactions? How did I feel after?

_____

_____

_____

_____

_____

_____

_____

_____

_____

_____

_____

_____

_____

_____

_____

_____

_____

_____

_____

_____

_____

Describe your natural object.

_____

_____

_____

_____

_____

_____

_____

Why did you choose it?

_____

_____

_____

_____

_____

_____

How does it make you feel?

_____

_____

_____

_____

_____

_____

_____

Draw It. Scribble It. Sketch It.

Emotions rarely get to be expressed freely without judgement or fear. Use this page to express your emotions—the good, the bad, the beautiful, the ugly. They all deserve to be seen. You deserve to be seen.

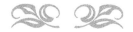

Week Two I AM

You may choose to walk in the same area or go somewhere else. If you are walking in a new area be sure to do a brief grounding and centering walking reflection before starting the I AM reflection. You have noticed the world and environment around you. Now it is time to reflect on who you are in your environment. The I AM reflection is meant to open your mind to the thought and affirmation that you are important in this world. Your thoughts, dreams, wants, and dislikes are important. You are important. Find a natural object to take back home with you. You may also use the same object from last week. **Alternative-**gentle stretches and simple chair or floor yoga.

Walking Reflection- As you walk observe the environment. The trees, grass, wildlife, and anything else that interests you. Listen even for cars and trains or planes flying overhead. Think about how these observations make you feel. Know that all these objects (living or non, natural or manmade) have a place. They have an intentional design. Know that you do as well. With eyes and palms open say the following to yourself.

Walking Affirmation

I AM here in this place, in this moment.

I AM present with myself and the Divine.

I AM one with myself and nature.

I AM intended.

I AM.

Walking Record

Length of Time <u>Distance</u>

_____

Date and Time

_____

> *Use your found object to do the Affirmation whenever you feel the need and you are indoors, this will keep you grounded to nature no matter where you are.*

Journal Reflection- What did I see on my walk that I did not notice before? How did I feel before I went on my walk? How did I feel after?

_____

_____

_____

_____

_____

_____

_____

_____

_____

_____

_____

_____

_____

_____

_____

_____

_____

_____

_____

_____

_____

_____

I Am Reflection- What new insights about myself do I now have? What do I like most about myself? How can I encourage these attributes?

_____

_____

_____

_____

_____

_____

_____

_____

_____

_____

_____

_____

_____

_____

_____

_____

_____

_____

_____

_____

_____

_____

_____

_____

Draw It. Scribble It. Sketch It.

Emotions rarely get to be expressed freely without judgement or fear. Use this page to express your emotions—the good, the bad, the beautiful, the ugly. They all deserve to be seen. You deserve to be seen.

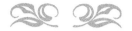

Week Three Choices

The decisions we make in life are not easy. Sometimes we must make on-the-spot choices that may have large consequences. Other times, there is time to think a decision through. There is time to weigh the pros and cons and to deliberate with others for their input. Big decisions can be a source of stress and anxiety. It is helpful to know that we can be guided through the decision-making process by our Higher Power if we give over the control. Let the outcome of well thought out decisions come in whatever form. Know that any choice leads to certain paths and not all paths are easy (some are uphill) even when the decision made was necessary or right. A choice is just that, a choice and once made the path must be followed until another choice can be made.

Walking Reflection- Try to quicken your pace a bit in sprints as you walk. If you are able, add in little jogs. This symbolizes the act of making a choice, the work involved in making that choice, and the outcome of the choice. Make your choice to jog or fast pace walk randomly. Notice how you choose when to do so. Notice how your body physically responds to your decision. Notice how your brain and mind responds to the decision. **Alternative-** Begin with gentle stretching. Move on to chair yoga you may choose to add a 2, 3, or 5 pound weight set for arm lifts (if you are able). Use the weights randomly, this will qualify as your sprint or jog.

Walking Affirmation

> I choose what is best given the information
> I have I have the right of choice
> I choose to choose

Walking Record

Length of Time <u>Distance</u>

_____

Date and Time

_____

> *You may choose another grounding object or continue to use the same one. If you choose to use a different one take time to notice any differences in reflection with this new object.*

Journal Reflection- What did I see on my walk that I did not notice before? How did I feel before I went on my walk? How did I feel after?

_____
_____
_____
_____
_____
_____
_____
_____
_____
_____
_____
_____
_____
_____
_____
_____
_____
_____
_____
_____
_____
_____
_____
_____

Choice Reflection- How did your body respond to the decision to jog or speed walk? How did you respond mentally? How did you respond emotionally? Did your response change over time? How?

_____

_____

_____

_____

_____

_____

_____

_____

_____

_____

_____

_____

_____

_____

_____

_____

_____

_____

_____

_____

_____

_____

_____

_____

Draw It. Scribble It. Sketch It.

Emotions rarely get to be expressed freely without judgement or fear. Use this page to express your emotions—the good, the bad, the beautiful, the ugly. They all deserve to be seen. You deserve to be seen.

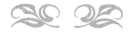

Week Four Acceptance

Whatt is acceptance? It is a word that is often heard in support groups and coaching sessions. In fact, the Serenity Prayer begins, "God, grant me the serenity to accept the things I cannot change". Acceptance, in psychological terms, "is a person's assent to the reality of a situation, recognizing a process or condition... without attempting to change it, protest, or exit." (Psychology Today, 2019) Our ability to accept the choices we make and their outcomes is what will carry us through tough times in life. Once we can accept what is, then we can look toward the future. Focusing intent on Acceptance resets our minds to not view situations and circumstances in our life negatively. They are just parts of the path that we walk, parts that are hard and trying. If we face these parts with acceptance, we come out on the other side stronger and understanding more about ourselves. We can face other challenges in life as opportunities for growth.

Walking Reflection This week, as you walk, focus on the most difficult parts of your route. Think about how you move through these parts of the trail or walking path. Feel the energy you exert as you go up a hill or incline. Feel the muscles in your legs, arms, and abdomen as you walk fast or jog or as you step over a rocky or muddy area. Accept that these challenges, inclines, mud, uneven parts on the path, are all a part of the journey. They are opportunities for physical growth. Observe small plants and trees. See where they grow. Look at how the root forces its way through concrete or the small plant pushes through the soil in a space it seems it should not be able to. **Alternative** continue chair or floor yoga and stretching as you do the above exercise.

Think about the obstacles to fitness you have; the many little (or big) things that get in the way of your exercise routine. Accept that these obstacles will arise. Accept that your response will not always be positive to these obstacles. Accept that there are days when you may not be able to get out and walk. Accept that you will not always make the right choice. Accept that this is okay. Accept that you are imperfect. A simple walking affirmation can be I Accept. No more. No less.

Walking affirmation

I Accept

Walking Record
Length of Time <u>Distance</u>

Date and Time

> Observe your nature object. How is it perfect? How is it imperfect? Do the imperfections change the way you feel about it? Can you accept that this object is perfect in its imperfection?

Journal Reflection- What did I see on my walk that I did not notice before? How did I feel before I went on my walk? Did I have any negative feelings or reactions? How did I feel after?

_____

_____

_____

_____

_____

_____

_____

_____

_____

_____

_____

_____

_____

_____

_____

_____

_____

_____

_____

_____

_____

_____

_____

_____

Acceptance Reflection- What things in my life do I find challenging? How can I work toward accepting these things without changing them? In what ways can I Accept my spouse? My children? Friends? Coworkers? Employers? Employees? In what ways can I Accept myself?

_____

_____

_____

_____

_____

_____

_____

_____

_____

_____

_____

_____

_____

_____

_____

_____

_____

_____

_____

_____

_____

_____

Draw It. Scribble It. Sketch It.

Emotions rarely get to be expressed freely without judgement or fear. Use this page to express your emotions—the good, the bad, the beautiful, the ugly. They all deserve to be seen. You deserve to be seen.

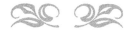

Week Five Change

This week we will look at change. Change is constant. It is cliché but true. As we learn to accept ourselves, others around us, and the circumstances we face, we begin to realize nothing is forever. The hard times come and go as well as the good times. I always thought of the saying "This too shall pass" to mean the negative stuff, the bad stuff, the hard stuff. Yet, it also refers to all the things we feel are good and right. Knowing this helps us accept situations without feeling an overwhelming sense of disappointment. It also helps us look for places where we can change our circumstance for the better. You have done so already. By starting this journey to connect to nature and yourself while at the same time working toward a healthier body, you have said to the universe I am a force of change!

Walking Reflection- Every step you take brings you closer to the mindset and health goal you wish to achieve. Notice how much stronger you are, how much more endurance you have. Take time also to notice the differences on your path. Notice how the leaves have shifted. Observe the feel of the air. If it was dry last time and now wet or the reverse notice how this difference feels. If you walk at different times of day observe the difference in light and shadow. Time changes all things, feelings, situations, places. Even the trees will grow tired by winter and shed their leaves for a well-deserved rest. They will change again in the Spring and again in the Summer. You too are changing. Every cell in your body is transforming. Your brain cells and synapses are forming new pathways, new connections that will transform your way of life forever.

Walking Affirmation

I am a force of change
I am a force of positive change
I can transform my life
One day, one step at a time

Walking Record

Length of Time <u>Distance</u>

_____

Date and Time

_____

> *Observe your nature object. How has it changed over time? Has it always looked this way?*
> *What has it endured to bring it to this moment? What experience can it give you?*

Journal Reflection- What did I see on my walk that I did not notice before? How did I feel before I went on my walk? How did I feel after?

_____

_____

_____

_____

_____

_____

_____

_____

_____

_____

_____

_____

_____

_____

_____

_____

_____

_____

_____

_____

_____

_____

_____

Change reflection- How has my life changed over the years? How have I reacted to that change? How can I react to change now? How can I guide positive change in my life moving forward? What is the best change I can make now and how will that improve my life?

_____

_____

_____

_____

_____

_____

_____

_____

_____

_____

_____

_____

_____

_____

_____

_____

_____

_____

_____

_____

_____

_____

Draw It. Scribble It. Sketch It.

Emotions rarely get to be expressed freely without judgement or fear. Use this page to express your emotions—the good, the bad, the beautiful, the ugly. They all deserve to be seen. You deserve to be seen.

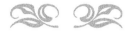

Week Six – The Path

You have walked a long road. You have reflected on your environment, your place in that environment. You have faced choices you make in everyday life and have begun to accept the beauty in the challenges you face. While you have done all this mental work you have increased your fitness and gained endurance. Look back at your journal and see your progress. Tally your time spent walking (or performing gentle workouts) over the last six weeks. Tally your distance. Take a moment to celebrate your new beginning.

This week we will focus on the paths we travel. It is hard to know where our choices will take us. In fact, it is impossible to know. All we can do is walk the path. We come to trust in the will of the Divine to guide us where we are meant to be. The key is staying on the path.

Walking Reflection Reflect on the path you travel on your walks. Pay attention to the way your body adjusts to change in the geography. Notice when you are able to walk the path almost without looking. Notice how you trust where the path leads and when it will end. Feel the familiarity of the path. Feel the peace that comes with acquaintance with your path. **Alternative** as you go through your routine of stretches and yoga and randomized weight lifting do the above activity.

Walking Affirmation

I trust the Divine to lead me my Path
I shall follow the Path set before me
I will stay the Path
I will not be distracted

Walking Record

Length of Time <u>Distance</u>

Hold your object and focus on the Path Affirmation. Remain grounded to nature. Remain focused on the path.

_____

Date and Time

_____

Journal Reflection- What did I see on my walk that I did not notice before? How did I feel before I went on my walk? How did I feel after?

_____

_____

_____

_____

_____

_____

_____

_____

_____

_____

_____

_____

_____

_____

_____

_____

_____

_____

_____

_____

_____

_____

_____

The Path Reflection- Where are you on your physical health journey? Where are you on your mental health journey? Where are you on your nature connection journey? What does the path forward look like now? What do you think it will look like in the next few weeks? How will you stay true to your journey?

_____

_____

_____

_____

_____

_____

_____

_____

_____

_____

_____

_____

_____

_____

_____

_____

_____

_____

_____

_____

_____

_____

Draw It. Scribble It. Sketch It.

Emotions rarely get to be expressed freely without judgement or fear. Use this page to express your emotions—the good, the bad, the beautiful, the ugly. They all deserve to be seen. You deserve to be seen.

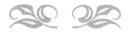

Congratulations!

You have completed your first steps to a healthier mind and body. I am honored you chose Nature Immersion for the Mind and Body as your beginner's path to health and wellness.

Are you ready to continue your journey of self-reflection and nature immersion? Are you ready to take your fitness and nutrition to the next level? It is my passion to help people connect with nature, God (Spirit/Universe, etc.), and themselves. I work with groups, individuals, couples, teens, and children.

Visit strongereveryday1111.com to learn more about my coaching programs, courses, excursions, and upcoming books.

Find me on the socials
FB @adventnature Ghene't Lee-Yong-Author
IG @healing_hikes_
IG @strongerveryday1111

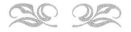

Acknowledgments

Thank you to Ruby Barnes, my magnificent editor, and to Shanda Trofe, my writing coach, for patience, guidance, and support through this process. Getting the ideas on paper is one thing. Having it make sense and look good is quite another!

CPSIA information can be obtained
at www.ICGtesting.com
Printed in the USA
BVHW072017051221
623292BV00014B/673

9 781087 980201